D0399677

SERENITY

SERENITY

Support and Guidance for People
with HIV, their Families, Friends,
and Caregivers

Paul Reed

SECOND EDITION

CELESTIAL ARTS
Berkeley, California

CELESTIAL ARTS
P.O. Box 7327
Berkeley, California 94707

Cover photograph by Martin Schweitzer
Cover design by Ken Scott
Author photo by David Lamm
Typography by Wilsted & Taylor, Oakland

Library of Congress Cataloging-in-Publication Data

Reed, Paul, 1956–
    Serenity: support and guidance for people with HIV, their families, friends, and caregivers / Paul Reed. — 2nd ed.
      p.   cm.
    Includes biobliographical references.
    ISBN 0-89087-604-5
    1. AIDS (Disease)—Psychological aspects.   2. AIDS (Disease)—Social aspects.   3. Homosexuality, Male.   I. Title.
RC607.A26R442   1990
362.1'9697'92—dc20   90-38097
                                                CIP

Manufactured in the United States of America

First Printing, 1987
Second Edition, 1990

1 2 3 4 5 — 91 90

CONTENTS

INTRODUCTION / ix

Chapter One / SERENITY / 1

Chapter Two / LONGING / 9

Chapter Three / MEMORY / 19

Chapter Four / AWAKENING / 27

Chapter Five / REALITY / 35

Chapter Six / SURRENDER / 45

Chapter Seven / TRANSFORMATION / 53

Chapter Eight / HOPE / 65

AFTERWORD / 77

POSTSCRIPT / 81

RESOURCES / 85

for Tom Gates,
in memory

INTRODUCTION

THESE essays chronicle one man's journey—my own—through the crippling fear of AIDS. After witnessing the crisis for six years, I realized that my life was shutting down. I was going numb trying to cope with what I read and saw daily, always trying to second guess the statistics. The "dispirit" I felt was overpowering. And I knew I somehow had to make peace with it, to find a positive way through the fear and back into the spirit of life I had once known.

The statistics and predictions are staggering. For those who have followed the AIDS crisis from the beginning or who are just now becoming aware, it can become almost impossible to comprehend what has happened as we go numb in self protection. And when we do stop to consider the magnitude of the tragedy, it seems crazy even to think of anything positive—what could possibly be positive in the midst of so much horror?

Well, the answer is nothing, necessarily. But for each of those statistics there are many people who, for whatever reasons, are survivors, and it is up to us to care for ourselves and our community by doing everything we can to move positively forward.

It is not easy to live with the threat of AIDS, whether

we're ill or well. It is not easy to live amidst the loss and dispirit, whether we're "threatened" or not. But it is imperative that we find the strength necessary to discover a way through it all.

Why? The temptation to despair is so strong that it can hardly be called a temptation. It just happens. In a sudden or gradual realization, we all come to a point where life seems robbed of spirit. And that is no way to live. The dispirit can be paralyzing on a personal level and on a community level. I have only to recall the powerful, loving surge of the spirit of *living* that I once felt to have my answer to the question of why it is necessary to discover a way through it all. We will not be able to turn the clock back, to imbue life with the meanings we once did, but I refuse to believe that fear and tragedy are stronger than courage and the vivid spirit to live. We cannot deny the horror, the dread, and the severe anger that this awful disease has brought about, but we can resolve to live as fully and richly as possible and to have as much, if not more, meaning in our lives than ever before.

In the first four chapters of this book, I discuss the experience of the AIDS epidemic within the gay community— what it's like for us to live with the stress of the epidemic, the kinds of problems we're encountering, the sorts of changes we're starting to make. Those chapters are very personal because it's important for all of us to know that we're not alone in this crisis, that many of us are going through the same tough times together. In the chapter "Reality," I discuss the importance of confronting plain facts so that you can take action, and the chapter "Surrender" shows some of the pitfalls and dangers that exist in trying to sort a way through it all—and how to avoid them. The final two chapters, "Transformation" and "Hope," give suggestions and examples of ways to make the best decisions for yourself about living well in the midst of the AIDS epidemic. At the end of the book is a chapter on Resources, where I recommend books that have been helpful to me, as well as phone numbers of organizations that can be of further guidance.

I hope that this book is helpful. I like to think of it as a "report from the front," as both a document of our times and a map for personal growth. I know what it is to live with the enormous stress of this epidemic, to try to decide what to do to maximize health, and I know what a difficult time it can be to find a way through it. By presenting these ideas and my own experiences, I hope it will be easier for others to find their best paths.

Chapter One

SERENITY

ABOUT the time we stopped saying "to die for" with regard to male beauty, a quiet revolution was under way. At the outset this health revolution was reluctant, the result of a tragic situation to which the only sane response was sudden, drastic change. Now we find ourselves in the midst of a new era, a time of difficult challenge.

It used to be that we wanted only the *image* of good health: tan, glowing skin, as if we had done nothing but sit on the beach all season; and, less specifically, we wanted an aura of vitality, a certain element of downright sexiness which some might call compulsive or hedonistic, but which was, truly, a spirit of readiness, as if one were willing to try *anything*, the sooner the better.

To achieve this we flocked by the thousands to those palaces of gay masculinity, our gyms. There we strained ourselves in an energetic frenzy that not only alleviated our childhood fears of athletic failure, but pumped our bodies into a masculine ideal. That frenzy felt like foreplay, so eager were we, so expectant of the glories yet to be in that time when every evening contained suspense and hopefulness.

I remember my first few months in the gym, when everything seemed new and exciting. Steam rising from the showers, small white terrycloth towels, the butch-jock sounds of metal clanking, men grunting, rock 'n' roll blasting from suspended speakers—all of it enthralled me and endeared me to that place where, at long last, beauty could be won.

Magazines of the day celebrated the new gay health consciousness in articles that linked the proliferation of gay bodybuilding with the health craze sweeping the country, though this connection was often complete nonsense. For did we not, all of us, know scores of friends who used drugs to energize their workouts, who smoked dope, took speed, and shot up anabolic steroids to facilitate that mad muscular frenzy?

I cared very little about real health back then, for I was young, fresh to the city, and filled with excitement over how much there was to do, how many people there were to be with, how much flesh there was. I wanted only Beauty, and what Nature had failed to supply, Iron would. Nutrition, relaxation, immunity—none of it mattered (or even occurred to us) in that optimistic push towards being a hunk.

And so, with profound self-discipline, we did what had to be done. Day after day, week upon week, we stoically, painfully entered that tabernacle of male perfection and did all those things one does there, sweating, dishing, waiting, hoping. It was a constant, mad press of thick bodies, all of us vibrating to Donna Summer and Sylvester, the same loud music that accompanied us later, long after the gym, when at the baths we put ourselves on display and waited to see if the effort would pay off.

HAVE they turned the music down in gyms? Or has our perception of exercise changed so much it seems as though the gyms are now quieter? One sometimes hearkens back to the "good old days" before AIDS, but memory often fails. We didn't enjoy perfect health even then, though we look back as if those were carefree days now lost. Have we forgotten hepatitis? Intestinal parasites? Gonorrhea?

The gyms are quieter now because their members are more sober about exercise and about life. The evolution of gay masculinity has taken us from our original place of bashful non-athleticism through that frenetic decade of muscles and disco, on into an era of transformation.

No longer does one hanker for the mere image of health; one is now utterly determined to achieve and keep the real thing. Because of the unpredictable nature of AIDS as well as the undeniable stress of life in these times, the goal now is a deep serenity bred by perfect balance, the peace of mind that manifests itself in a relaxed, fluid body and a rich, hearty soul.

Image is still important, but now we want a new image, the image of perfect health. To this end we have responded with psychology and fashion. We have developed an aversion to wearing the kind of clothes—or in any way projecting an image—that might suggest the old feeling of ready sexiness. Much of the conformity that earned us the name "clones" is gone. Tight jeans torn and tattered at pressure points, t-shirts a size too small, colored jockstraps, bomber jackets, tight red plaid shirts, motorcycle boots, bandanas— these are now found fluttering in the breeze at sidewalk sales, or one stumbles across them while rummaging in the dark recesses of dresser drawers or in dusty boxes stuck together in forgotten closet corners.

Fashion victims abound, for nothing communicates an image of newness more readily than the "latest" attire. And being a little fat—just the slightest hint of a roll about the waistline—is also a desirable trait. The painful thinness of yesteryear's disco bunnies has yielded to the desire for meatiness, for a man whose appearance bespeaks an appetite for *life*.

We sometimes still see the old practitioners, though in far fewer numbers—still working out too hard, a lost expression on their faces as they rest between exercises, as if unable to snap out of the broken promise; serenity has yet to be learned. But the new gay male, in his loose, relaxed fashions, strolls along the street with an expression of calm, a smile ready when his eyes meet another's (no more the hard frown of heavy cruising), his determination for good health and peace of mind an absolute aura.

To achieve serenity we still flock by the thousands to the gyms—those palaces of gay masculinity—but we have enriched our health regimens with many new elements. Serenity is induced when we achieve balance among these many elements.

For strength and physical proportioning we continue to pump iron, swelling muscles into their desired shapes, chiselling thighs, adding bulk here and there, and increasing overall body strength. For endurance, energy, and inner health we add aerobics to our daily plan by bicycling, swimming, running, or aerobics classes. We do yoga or stretching for flexibility and balance.

For nutrition and freedom from addiction we review our diets, eliminating the things that rob us of energy, things like sugar, caffeine, and simple carbohydrates. We limit drinking, virtually eliminate drugs, and completely forbid smoking.

Rest becomes essential, and it's composed of several things—a good night's sleep, of course, as well as moments of meditation or simple silence when we create time for ourselves to be alone, to quiet all the psychic interference of our daily life. Such quiet moments create the real appreciation of serenity, because in being still we truly *feel* the calm of a healthy body. Where tension, fear, worry, and judgment once reigned, now taking their place are peace, acceptance, and gentleness.

Later, when after all of this we retire to bed and lie thinking in the dark, we remember everything we have done and all the changes we have made. And, with a peaceful but plain sense of relief at having left the tensions of the day behind us, we drift off to sleep as we calculate the odds and always hedge our bets: we will do everything we can to survive.

OUR priorities, then, have shifted. Now we require much more than just the appearance of health. We must have the real thing, a sound mind and healthy soul in a strong body. That classical goal is now ours, and events have catapulted us forward at a dizzying rate. Where we once aspired to a healthy glow, we now desire glowing health.

This represents more than a quest for good health, more than a desire to avoid illness, more than a wish for a long life. This shift toward serenity symbolizes a profound transition—we are abandoning materialism and embracing spirituality.

Now, this is no minor shift. For too long, gay people have been denied spiritual access, if you will. Organized religion has shunned the gay man and lesbian, shutting us out completely and turning us away from the deeper realities those religions represent—tranquillity, faith, hope, courage, love, and acceptance.

Instead we embraced materialism and physical culture with a vengeance, heaping high value on possessions, beauty, the shape of a face, the feel of muscle. There is nothing wrong with this—materialism has as its ultimate goal to provide comfort, to make this life passage easier and more enjoyable. But as we all know, physical satisfaction can be empty. So here we are on the cutting edge of a new social revolution, demonstrating in our fight against disease and our quest for calmness of mind and spirit that real happiness is won by the heart.

Now, there is always a problem when using the term "spiritual." The word has gooey connotations—things like church or temple, or worse yet, all that touchy-feely business we associate with "feeding our souls" or "raising our consciousness." What I mean here has a little to do with all of that, yes, but what I really mean has to do with finding harmony in life—accepting things as they are, being nice to people, not being self-centered but giving, and always looking forward to the future without dwelling on the hurtful past. These require effort, constant and slow, and that effort—and the good feelings it promises—are a large part of what spirituality is all about.

Of course it runs deeper as well. We all know the feeling of connectedness with nature and humankind, that feeling we humorlessly call "in tune with the universe." It is really a matter of being quiet—keeping still in order to hear one's own thoughts and feelings—and of keeping one's attitude toward life on a positive, hopeful track, filled with that forgiveness and simple acceptance we learn in silence.

As the saying goes, there are many paths to the top of the mountain, and so we come to this spirituality from many angles. The important point is that we have come to it and that it has colored our values and the quality of life in a significant way. What a relief it is finally to look at each other—even in the midst of such tragedy—as just human beings, gentle men with feelings, all of us struggling as best we can.

What, then, has changed? Gay men continue to come out of their closets, migrate to gay urban centers, and lead lives in that legendary pursuit of happiness. An edge has been lost, a certain tension is now gone, but it is being replaced by the enriching experience of redefining "community." Survival is the order of the day, and we're doing everything we can to ensure it—from meditation to angry protest, from early intervention to the fight for better treatment, for equal rights, for the opportunity to lead healthy lives.

Chapter Two

LONGING

YEARS ago I moved to San Francisco to escape three elements of life—loneliness, isolation, and longing. These had been the moods of childhood, the long-suffering trial inflicted on many gay youngsters: an early awareness of singularity and difference that can become isolation and pain before, finally, asserting itself as individuality. Adolescence unfolded not as some wonderful playground of discovery or the usual process of dating, going steady, attending the prom. Rather, those teenage years were a proposition of unendurable yearning, impatience to be free of the boundaries of family, hometown, school—in short, to be free of conventionality.

I remember how, during those adolescent years, when I dreamt of escape, I dreamt not of San Francisco, but of New York. New York was the symbol—the sum—of everything that I would become. Sometimes late at night I would catch a portion of the Johnny Carson show, the guests so sophisticated and elegantly dressed, their cigarettes sending up arrogant spirals of smoke, their laughter decadent and indifferent, and I felt that eventually I would go to New York, where, with all these other urban sophisticates, I would fully realize my destiny as a member of some sardonic set.

It was to San Francisco I eventually came, and the loneliness, longing, and isolation never completely dissipated. The sweeping vistas of distant hills and waters only deepened those feelings of longing, for everywhere I looked, there was somewhere else to be, far off. Other cities—with their towers or rich houses snuggled into hills—could always be seen for some way, reminding me of things yet to be had, yet to be done. Once, when my mother came to visit me in the city, I spent several days feeling exactly as I had when I was trapped by my family in adolescence, a feeling recorded perfectly by Edmund White in *A Boy's Own Story*: "All around me—at the post office where we had a box, in the general store, on docks, sailboats and water skis—young people with iodine-and-baby-oil tans, trim bodies and faultless teeth were having fun." While shopping with Mother one of those days during her visit, I felt that the dozens of beautiful young men we passed were completely beyond reach, just as they had been throughout childhood. I stared at one exceptional man who held my gaze, but the ritual was cut short when my mother asked my opinion about the possibility of inserting a Dr. Scholl's foot pad into the pair of navy pumps she had just purchased at Magnin.

Escape from the feeling of being a misfit as a gay youngster in a simple country town—this was the essence of longing in childhood and young adulthood. For my family lived not far from San Francisco, in a hot town beside the Sacramento River. Yet the City—as San Francisco is called by the neighboring provincials—was completely beyond my reach, for it was as if I were forever trapped within the confines of an unsophisticated life. At fifteen and sixteen, my sister and I would visit the City, take boxes at the Curran Theatre, observe Jean Simmons, Margaret Hamilton, Deborah Kerr, Katharine Hepburn as they acted upon the stage. Yet I was vividly aware that the gap between theatre and real life was as large as that between my dreams of freedom and the plainness of my life. Afterwards we would walk Union Square or Post Street, and my eyes would wander, this time inquisitive as they met with the eyes of men who passed within inches of my teenage body.

S UCH longing is an integral part of the gay experience, an emotional response to life's circumstances that brings great pain throughout childhood and beyond. A friend once angrily asked me if I honestly thought that longing was the province of gay people, didn't I think that straight people, too, sat beside the window and yearned for distant places, for other times, for the past? I answered that of course they did, but that for me, longing had been more than a passing mood, more than something in which I had occasionally wallowed. Longing had been the *central* experience of adolescence, and the things that I had hoped would quell it—love, hedonism, sex, availability, anonymity, adulthood in general—never did.

It was then that I surmised that longing is integral to those of us who have been spiritually deprived by a society which denies us the food for our souls and hearts. Gay people are groomed for longing by the very fact of the lack of a place for gay people within society. Gay people do not fit in. There is no place provided for us, no special role into which we can step, at least no special role into which we would want to step. Everywhere we look—television, billboards, magazines, wherever—we are reminded, if not completely consciously, that we are not allowed a real, viable place in society. This is not a new message, of course. This is the central message of the gay political movement, as well as its central goal—to create viability, to mold society into a new image that more closely reflects the reality of its members.

But it is also the central foundation for longing and for the spiritual crisis that a life of longing can precipitate. The larger, prevailing society does not reflect the reality of gay experience. We *know* that we are here, that we are productive, that we love, that our lives can be as viable as anyone else's. But what we know is not common knowledge. Our experience—our existence—is not generally known or accepted. We are denied the depth of our own existence because society does not acknowledge our existence. And so we long for things to be different, we wish that life were easier. We wish that we could marry each other or live freely, openly; we wish we could behave exactly as we feel, with no need to hide, no need to be discreet about whom we love—all with the acknowledgement, recognition, blessing, and support of society: of our families, friends, ministers, rabbis, doctors, teachers—everyone who touches our lives.

Now many of us work toward establishing this acceptance and recognition. In the last twenty years, we have been working very hard to win the support of society, to help teach those around us that society is made up of more than one kind of individual, that all members of society are unique, filled with wonderful, obvious and subtle differences.

The subtle differences of gay people have intrigued me for a long time. We are kind and gentle people. We are a loving community from which violence does not readily erupt. But it is this difference of spirit—this *kindness* of spirit—that also feeds longing, for the schism between this loving mode of our community and the rough mode of a world we want to remake can be profound. We wish that things were very different; we long for them to be otherwise, on a spiritual as well as physical plane, just as we longed for different surroundings and attitudes as gay children and teenagers coping hopelessly in a foreign land.

This is not a haughty proposition of "moral superiority," nor is it one that presumes a bias against people who don't lead gay lifestyles, for surely the world is filled with loving nongays who, too, long for social change (though I have always wondered about a certain question here—do we seek social change and spiritual serenity because we are gay, or are we gay because we seek social and spiritual change?)

For a terrible time we have been thrown into a spiritual transition by the health crisis. The good news is that our experience of longing has always been our spiritual catalyst, and the confrontation of the health crisis has oriented us more strongly toward the deeply caring modes to which we had always leaned, if not achieved. After the hedonistic rush of the seventies we are rapidly moving into an era of giving, selfless love, caring, and self-responsibility. We are nurturing our souls as fully as we can—a task we had always done, even in the mad rush—for nonconformity and peaceful rebellion always arise from a basis of love and longing for betterment.

Many of us have died, so we have not all been given an opportunity in this transformation of spirit, this solution to the crisis of longing. That is tragic, and there is certainly no way to make good sense of it. It would seem that to look for a silver lining in the cloud of the AIDS crisis would be an act of folly. But the solution to longing (if one would seek to escape its sanguine grip) is to take action. And taking action always brings about change—internal and external. The trick is in recognizing longing for what it really is—a spiritual crisis that calls out for action. The next trick is to *accept* the challenge as the catalyst for change and to determine that by seeking change we are also seeking growth, not just destruction.

WHAT does any of this have to do with the health crisis in which we now find ourselves? Haven't we seen that there is terrible tragedy here, that the way of growth and change is fraught with horrendous setbacks? Of course we cannot erase the death we have seen, the loss we have suffered. Of course we cannot cavalierly disregard the mounting numbers and fear we all face—sick or well.

But we *can* recognize that a powerful ingredient in determining the course of any eventuality is the level of work that we are willing to put into our personal growth. But we must always remember that personal growth is not a talisman, not a magical charm; it is simply what we must do in order to move ahead as human beings.

Yet the very thought of moving ahead is becoming increasingly anathema to many of us, for the future appears at best as a grim fog on a shadowed marsh, at worst as nonexistent. We wish to turn back the hands of the clock, not move forward. When epidemiologists tell us that such-and-such a number of people are expected to die within five or ten years, it is terribly difficult to arise in the morning and face the future with enthusiasm. Who cares about personal growth when every day the newspapers hand out virtual death sentences? Who can give a damn whether the gay community lives or dies when the pressures of possibly imminent illness make one feel like cowering under the covers or fleeing to the hills? Of what possible use is "personal growth" at a time like this?

These are the questions of despair. Hopelessness is a common and widespread ailment. And so we allow ourselves to stall, to slow down or halt our personal growth, because it would seem that there is nothing to grow into. It would seem that our community is becoming increasingly fractured and useless, that there is no reason for self-improvement, for spiritual nourishment, for emotional maturity.

The demands of a crisis are the demands of growth. Now more than ever we each require strength of character, emotional stability, and nourished souls that are ready to give what friends, lovers, and community demand of us: help, hope, encouragement. It is the same demand that has always been created by longing—the demand to change things, to improve one's lot in life. The blandness of longing is nothing compared to the knife-sharp pain of the AIDS epidemic, and so our response must be equal to the task.

We have to overcome the temptations of escape—nostalgia, denial, refusal, hardness of heart, bad habits, and hopelessness—to turn away from the window of longing and its melancholy view.

Chapter Three

MEMORY

MEMORY can play a dirty trick on us. It can render past experiences as the most blissful and peaceful of times. It can select only the very best—and eliminate the worst or even the slightly shoddy.

In the midst of a crisis like AIDS—where our entire focus has shifted, our old world has fallen away—we are strongly tempted to dredge up old memories and play with them like childhood teddy bears. They comfort us, reminding us that no, we haven't missed out, we *were* there, we *did* enjoy it.

This can be a healthy indulgence, or it can be a foul trap. It depends on the approach. To settle oneself comfortably with a cup of tea and reminisce, to sit cozily in a booth at the cafe with friends and remember, to open the trunk of fun times past and handle those memories with fondness can be momentarily satisfying and enriching.

But to become obsessed with the past—to feel that the best times are over, to do nothing but yearn for a time that has come and gone and will never return—can render life meaningless and moody.

It is true that we in the gay community—women and men—created and lived through one of the most exciting periods of social and sexual transformation in recent history. The period that gay people call "post-Stonewall" (because it followed the 1969 riots at the Stonewall bar in New York City, the first time that gay people fought back against authority and laid claim to our right to be as we are) was a tremendous time of general cultural upheaval throughout the western world, not only in terms of sexual freedom, gay and straight, but in terms of liberalizing attitudes in general. After 1969 (after "Stonewall") gay people came out of their closets *en masse* throughout the United States and western Europe and declared that we were tired of hiding, of suffering, of living our lives without the fullness of love.

And so was born the "Gay Liberation Movement" amid the sexual revolution of the late sixties and early seventies. Those were exciting times, times of rich experimentation and the forging of an entirely new set of social and sexual practices. And no one would deny that those were rich times, that something amazing and even magical went on.

But it was a *different* time than the present, and to look backwards—to whine that things are not as they were—is simply an exercise in frustration that accomplishes nothing. Scrutinizing the past cannot alter what has happened, and clinging to romantic memories of halcyon days can lead in only one direction. It is the downward path, leading away from growth, away from strength, leading only to disharmony, frustration, and lack of vitality.

We have adopted all manner of reference to our past sexual freedom: "The Good Old Days" is a common phrase. Sometimes we hear people refer to "B.A."—as in "Before AIDS." And of course, the more direct references: "The Sleazy Days;" or, "When We Used to Have Fun."

There is an honest element in this nostalgia, this yearning for the past, because those *were* good times, unusual times, a once-in-a-lifetime kind of experience. It is one of the great ironies of this crisis that what we most urgently longed to do back then was what most urgently challenged us to growth. We acted out of love and enthusiasm for ourselves and for our community. And while this may now sound something like an apology, it is nothing of the sort. It is, in fact, a wise thing for us to remember—as society tries so desperately to lay blame and create guilt—that at the time, it seemed we had a calling to establish a new order of relations, or, at least, a viable *alternative* form of relations. We were forging a camaraderie, a brotherhood, a sisterhood, a community of like-minded women and men interwoven within the larger society.

And now, the irony—what seems a dirty trick—is that those new relations, as we expressed it in that exuberant, free sexuality, seem to have backfired. But it is important to remember that it only *seems* to have backfired. For it was not the forging of new relations that caused the health crisis. It was not the alternative sexuality or the alternative love relationships that brought AIDS about. AIDS was brought about by the introduction of a virulent microbe, a disease.

So, the challenge to continue our valuable role as forgers of alternative relationships is considerably more complex than we ever could have imagined in that time of long nights and sweet strangers.

There can be more to this problem of memory than nostalgia, though, more than just a simple hearkening to halcyon days of a bygone, "golden era." A friend of mine recently confided that he was suffering from what he called an "affliction of memory." He couldn't stop *remembering*. He would be walking down the street, or shopping in a store, or driving in his car when all of a sudden he would be filled with the most vivid memory of doing the very same things when he first moved to the City. It wasn't an experience of *deja vu*. It was more a deep, bittersweet feeling that re-called—for a fleeting moment—the exact mood, the exact thoughts and feelings that he had had in the same places in 1979 or 1980.

What was painful to him about it was the deep feeling of longing, a sad, almost overwhelming feeling of just how en-thusiastic and joyous his life had seemed in those days. He was re-experiencing all the eagerness of looking forward to a night at the baths or a weekend of revelry. And whenever he felt like that, he remembered just how cathartic those experiences had been. His present-day troubles would fall away in those moments of sharp memory—and he would recall just how the experience of going to the baths or clubs had put life's problems in perspective. It was the loss of that escape valve that made these memories so vivid and so bit-ter.

He was very troubled by these experiences, and was con-sidering seeing a counselor about them. He spoke to me about them in nearly a whisper one rainy Saturday. I thought about it for quite a while as he described his expe-riences in detail. I had felt the very same way on occasion, but had merely dismissed it as nostalgia. But as I listened to his detailed—and obviously sad—description of the all-consuming nature of these experiences, of how they seemed to him to be nearly "time-travel" moments, I suspected that there was something in it of the loss of innocence.

He did see a counselor about it, eventually, and what she told him confirmed my suspicion—that he was feeling more than nostalgia, that he was going through an experience that comes to most everyone at some point in life.

My friend was aware of such a turning point in life. But what made it so much more vivid and painful for him was that it was forced on him by the AIDS crisis. Without it, his loss of innocence might have been an experience of several years, simply a maturing process that would have come with age. Instead, it was something that descended without warning and, more importantly, without the proper maturity, age, or accumulation of experience to deal with it naturally. It was that suddenness—and lack of control—that was making him suffer emotionally.

As gay youngsters, many of us were denied what might be called an appropriate adolescence. Psychologists and writers have repeatedly drawn metaphors between the frantic sex-crazed days of the early gay liberation movement and teenage adolescence. The idea here is that the gay community was collectively experiencing the adolescence that we were denied because, of course, as gay teenagers we didn't fit in. We weren't allowed to participate in the dating rituals and sexual experimentation that would have befitted our desires. We either skipped the experience altogether or else we did it in a way that wasn't really ours—taking on girlfriends when we would have preferred boyfriends, re-sorting to locker-room masturbation scenes when we would have loved a back-seat smooch with one of the guys.

Of course, drawing such metaphors is often unproductive, because in the first place every individual is different. To suggest that we—millions of us—experienced the same thing—that can now be labelled a collective adolescence—is a bit farfetched. And in the second place, if we did experience a collective adolescence, so what? We're not experiencing adolescence now, and if some of us perchance need to, then we will; we'll find a safe way to be adolescents again.

In the present moment, in the plain light of a reality that contains fear and ugliness, such ruminations can lead to despair, if we let them. They are an unproductive diversion. That is why we must have clear minds and healthy memories. For if we are to rise to the work that must be done, if we are to preserve our community and our relations in this time of great emotional and physical upheaval, we must not let our minds wander into traps of romanticized memories or deluded nostalgia. We must not despair.

Is there any benefit in remembering? Must we—as this line of thinking might suggest—block all memory of the glory days of our sexual freedom? Must we stop remembering and simply exist in the present moment?

Well, the present moment is always a wonderful place to be, for it is all that we ever really know or have. But memories can play a positive role in our lives. Just as another individual would never pretend that he had not had an ad-olescence (can one imagine blocking memories of high school prom night, or cold weekends tucked cozily in the grandstands at the school football game?), neither must we quash these memories, these feelings that rise up whenever we recall the early days.

Rather, we can imagine them to be the fertile ground upon which we are building a strong and deeply interwoven community. We can experience these memories as vivid snapshots in our photo album, full of life, color, energy, and cheer. We cannot take them as the standard against which we measure the present, but rather as the contribution to the future that history always represents.

We can see how far we have come, how deeply we are feeling life right now. These memories are a part of us—the only vivid part of the past that remains with us. Paradise is not lost. Paradise is within each of us.

Chapter Four

AWAKENING

O N sunny Saturdays there used to be a certain rhythm to the day. As restless as the breeze drafting the curtains wide, I would get up mid-morning, turn on the hot water in the shower, turn this way and that in front of the mirror to examine the payoff of effort at the gym. Steam poured through the transom as I showered and felt a sense of pure peace under the hot water. Then, after towelling, I'd scramble eggs and pull on tight clothes.

Outside, the warmth of spring or autumn enveloped me as I walked along those city streets of jazz and noise to reach the Muni Metro. And when I next emerged into fresh air I saw hundreds of beautiful men nearly dancing in the street, Castro Street, a defiant, naked celebration of denied male beauty, now wantonly jumping for joy.

It was dreamlike, even then, as if we had made a long descent into the glories of the unconscious. It seems even more like a dream now, because things have happened to pinch us awake.

Yet that rhythmic life of sunny weekends and long nights had been an awakening in itself. We had awakened from the darkness of closets, from the shadows of oppression and fear, from the ignorance of the absolute rightness of what we were, what we wanted, and what we eventually went out and seized as our rightful own. We had awakened from lives of conformity, from lies and whispers, and together we had forged those new relations, that consciousness we called gay community. That we would come to regard that time of awakening as a time of dreaming is a curious twist of fate. When we were startled awake—are we still dreaming?—the sudden rush of madness made any option seem rather grim.

Have Saturdays changed all that much? The rigors of chores still loom, but those half-naked afternoons and naked nights have vanished. Again we whine: It's not like it used to be. And the complaint is sympathetically noted. After all, we didn't choose to abandon that fun. We didn't choose this cruel reality. We were forced by circumstance to take a different path.

At first we hoped it would be only a detour. Time and statistics have proven it was not. We have been forced into a new world which seems strangely fearful, overwhelming at times. And it has been a painful, emotional maze of uncertainty, panic, curious longings, and quiet moments alone with worries about the future.

None of us would deny the pain that awakening to the AIDS crisis has brought. No one could possibly say "Well, it doesn't worry me, I've hardly thought about it." The uncertainty is with us every day, and as things around us worsen, we often feel adrift in life, wondering if the promise of the future that we once simply took for granted will be broken.

Broken promises—that is one of the strongest feelings we have. For those who have not fully awakened to the reality of AIDS, or for those who have learned (and so easily) to push that reality to the backs of our minds, life can be filled with a sense of broken promise so strong that we operate in a dim half-world of hopeless expectancy, like travelers awaiting a flight delayed far too long. And that is not an easy way to live.

Beyond the disturbing feeling of broken promise is the fear that comes with being a member of the group that is defined as being at highest risk for contracting AIDS. To live each day with that possibility places us in a severe stress situation. It is not unlike the kind of stress that concentration camp inmates experienced during World War II, as, each day, they awaited the "daily selection." The stress of thus "living under the sword" can approach intolerable levels. And that, too, is not an easy way to live.

Most of us have been forced out of sexual frenzy and carefree play into the harsh reality that this crisis is very real, and that it is going to be with us for a very long time. Some have used this forced awareness as a scapegoat, excusing our depressions and cynicism with statistics and news analyses that read like hysterical nightmares.

But some are finding a different path, a voluntary path, turning toward reality and its bizarre twists and walking straight into it, saying: "Alright, things are bad, there's no denying that, but I intend to survive this mess, to accept its fears as a problem to be overcome. I intend to do everything

I can to weather this storm—change my outlook, my habits, whatever it takes."

ONE does not arrive at such a clear, logical, "problem-solving" approach easily. But again, there are many paths on the mountain, and it doesn't really matter precisely which path we take. But facing reality, the willful confrontation with the fear headlong—this is something that happens voluntarily, when one decides to do it. If the decision is not made—if we do not sit down and say "Okay, this is it, from now on I'm taking steps to deal with this"—very little inner growth is possible. But when the confrontation is taken on, the voluntary turn toward a state of inner peace and serenity is a miracle.

And it's a miracle precisely because it is the only one that leads out of the paralysis of fear. And, interestingly, it is also the simplest path, for with the conscious decision to follow it comes enormous relief by letting go of the tension of fear. And letting go of tension—that relief—is invigorating.

BUT , unfortunately, awakening is too often an experience of sudden, crippling fear—a terror that does not remit. This is the hard part. It's one of the reasons we would rather not move towards awakening. Who in his right mind would choose to open his eyes to pain and catastrophe?

Pain, catastrophe, fear, terror . . . these are harsh words

for harsh realities. Using them comes strangely close to sensationalism, to stirring up panic, mimicking the preachers of fear and the doomsayers who daily create paranoia in the gay and straight media.

But if there is one all important fact to understand about this challenge—this appeal to inner strength that the AIDS crisis engenders—it is that nobody would try to make light of it. Nobody would suggest that it is not a terrible tragedy, that we wish we had never heard the word, that if we could turn the clock back we would. Nobody would suggest that being *forced* onto a track of personal growth is the best way to embark on a journey to inner strength.

No, that would be insanity, another way to deny the cold simplicity of tragedy. Life is tough. Everyone seems to agree about that. And AIDS is a dreadful tragedy. No argument there. So, of course, awakening from the past, and looking at the AIDS crisis without blinders has *got* to be a tough, painful experience.

Of course the ideal way to embark on a new path of personal growth would be to come to it from one's own inner life, from one's own innate hunger for meaning and relationship. But that kind of awakening has not been a tradition among gay people, because we have been cut off from the traditional routes of spiritual challenge. And the non-traditional routes that we explored—new relationship forms, physical sexuality to the point of ecstasy and catharsis, completely new and unique formulations of ideology and politics—have now, in part, been rendered defunct by the completely new set of circumstances that the AIDS crisis has precipitated.

So, we are abruptly awakening to a spiritual journey by being *forced* into it by outside circumstances. The fact that it has been forced, rather than found, is not as important as the fact that the challenge is there, that we are aware of it, that we accept it, and that we are moving on.

Chapter Five

REALITY

R EALITY can be harsh. Much of life—work, shopping, laundry, cleaning, budgeting, running errands, waiting in line—is, quite simply, tedious. The tedium can be downright painful in its consequent boredom. And so we learn, from an early age, to escape into imagination as a relief from all this painful boredom. This imaginative escape valve—with its resultant fantasies and behaviors—has allowed us ample room in which to avoid anything that is too painful to think about. We can simply invent reasoning or diversions.

We never seem to stop making things up—from simple daydreaming to elaborate projections about our lovers, employers, and the world at large. And while on the one hand the imaginative process is the foundation for art and is, in large part what distinguishes humans from the rest of the animal kingdom, the great problem with all this myth-making is that it obscures our perception of reality—of what is really going on, in the concrete, physical, down-to-earth realm.

It can be difficult to live in the real world, to sit still long enough to examine what is really happening and to distinguish that from what is simply the imaginative "film" through which we are viewing events in our lives and in the world around us.

Living in reality is a task—it is something that has to be worked at, daily. If we have learned to avoid a great deal of reality through habit, it can be harder to grasp reality than if we have always striven for a realistic view.

But living in reality is a worthwhile goal, for only then can we see what is truly going on around us, and only then can we adequately and clearly evaluate the situations and crises in which we find ourselves.

And only then, finally, can we be free of the pain—the anxiety and mental anguish—that accompanies habitual misperception.

B UT living in reality requires effort—to overcome the seductive strength of our imaginative defenses. In large part, to live in reality means to accept things as they are. And accepting things as they are is one of the hardest challenges in life.

Reality is strong medicine. It is a way of life, a way of looking at the world and its events that is both potent and effective. There are many ways that we can learn to live realistically, and each of us must—if we are to accept the challenge to live well—learn how to do it. For many, living realistically involves study and thought. For others, counseling or professional therapy might be the best route. Or, most easy is to begin to exercise your "reality faculties," to train yourself to adopt the habit of evaluating what is going on in terms of physical and emotional fact.

It is almost a matter of "reading between the lines," or rather, reading *beyond* the lines. For most "lines" come couched in one meaning or another—laden with the mantel of interpretation, prevailing ideas, and habits of thinking that pervade the culture in which we live. When you're living fully in reality, it feels almost like intuition, because the best, clearest thought simply "comes" to you, as if what you're hearing, reading, or being told is slightly off the mark. You develop the facility—which, in time, becomes a habit—of examining the actual facts of any situation, seeing what really is happening in plain action and then, of evaluating the possible meaning for yourself and for others.

SOMETIMES the way in which we understand reality can be another myth in itself. That is the problem with interpreting an approach to AIDS. The realities of pain, suffering, disfigurement, public apathy that amounts to hateful complicity, and death are so grim that, of course, we choose to avoid them, though that choice is often unconscious.

We have many ways to shield ourselves from a realistic appraisal of the AIDS crisis. We can simply block out all thoughts of it—just suppress any thought or image that comes to mind—though this would be nearly impossible nowadays, with the constant barrage of upbeat histrionics in the media. We can contrive paranoid theories about the origin of the virus and its spread—notions about AIDS as deliberate germ warfare or as a dreadful, hushed-up mistake of genetic engineering. Or, we can focus on a single aspect of the overall picture, perhaps constantly rehashing thoughts about funding or miracle cures or the complex politics of the situation, without ever confronting the sad reality of a friend in need or the fears that come and go.

There is afoot a movement to interpret AIDS as a call to arms, or, as this book might seem to suggest at first glance, as a challenge to spiritual growth. Such interpretations—positive though they may be—can also be myths of denial. One cannot simply say, "Well, now, let's see . . . AIDS is a call to inner growth, so that's how I'm going to think of it from now on"—and think that one has confronted reality and chosen a "higher path." All these notions—of higher paths, spiritual challenges, and so on—can be methods by which to deny the AIDS crisis as effectively as any other form of denial.

Which doesn't mean that the challenge to spiritual growth isn't a *part* of the meaning of the AIDS crisis, or that to find the most positive path through the crisis isn't both a laudable and highly practical approach. It simply cannot be seen as the big picture.

Along this same line is the popular theory emerging from the holistic health movement which suggests that AIDS is really a sickness of the spirit, that mental and emotional attitudes are the culprits here, that the oppression of gays and minorities pre-dispose them to disease. In its crudest form, this theory attributes responsibility for disease to the individual who is sick—who brought the illness on himself by bad attitudes and unhealthy living.

This argument is frightfully close in spirit to the fundamentalist Christian interpretation of AIDS, which sees AIDS as God's punishment for wicked living. Both arguments attribute ultimate responsibility—and *cause*—to the individual. Sin, deviation from God's plan, and immorality are Christianity's conceptual parallels to holistic health's accusations of failure to meditate, losing touch with nature, and self-pollution through refusal to follow strict diets.

In its most sophisticated form, however, the holistic health theory sees attitude as merely setting the stage for *susceptibility* to disease, and this lies much closer to what allopathic medical practitioners and clinicians have already observed, that there are beliefs and attitudes which result in certain behaviors—such as neglecting good nutrition or failing to exercise or simply always maintaining a high level of stress—that then predispose an individual to a weakened physical constitution, which might lead to the eruption of a condition. But the link is indirect, and it is simply unfair and uncompassionate to attribute a person's condition willy-nilly to his emotional status.

All of this suggests that sorting one's way through a personal interpretation of AIDS has become akin to picking a religion to which to convert. The complexity of the issue—from biology and medicine to sexuality and responsibility, to ethics, politics and civil liberties, to funding and family matters and patient care—demands a complex interpretation.

But, a complex interpretation is never what we, as fun-loving, simple human beings, *want*. It is neither easy nor comforting to deal with anything in a complicated way. But realistic approaches to life's problems often require that we, quite plainly, grapple with several converging issues at once, and that we accept and try to become comfortable with the fact that there is often no simple answer. Too often we wish there were more simple answers in life, and we carry the hope for a simple answer in our hearts like a great beacon. We hope for a talisman.

It can be highly comforting, however, to realize that complexity is the order of the day, that the only realistic approach to AIDS is bound to be complicated, confusing, and time-consuming. It can be highly comforting to know that if you feel confused, anxious, and burdened with knowledge you wish you'd never gained, then you are, in fact, dealing with AIDS in the only realistic way there is.

Many people find the stress of living with the threat of AIDS to be too great, nearly unbearable. It is hard not to know if and when you might contract the disease. If you know that you are sero-positive for the AIDS virus, it can be doubly hard to live your life in a positive manner, for the constant worry of syptomatic eruption is a tremendous drain. And if you are living with an Aids-Related Condition (ARC), the impatience for a resolution to your condition can be incredibly stressful, preoccupying your every thought, even pushing you into a wish to contract the full disease and be done with it.

This is normal. This is living "under the sword." And it is simply the way that things are. Perhaps the hardest lesson to learn is that of acceptance—there is no easy answer, the stress is nearly intolerable, and there is no turning back.

A friend of mine who has always been a student of history once told me that a study of world history yields always the same conclusion: that things happen, things that no one planned or wanted, things like epidemics, wars, atrocities. This, unfortunately, is part of life, but we tend, probably too often, to lull ourselves into false security with physical luxury and the promises of the future that we interpret our childhood to have given us.

But the plain fact is that we don't always get what we want. Things happen—good and bad—and we have to learn over and over again to accept them as they happen. Surely the horror and the atrocious reality of the Holocaust should prove that things just happen, things much worse than anyone could ever have imagined.

Without stretching the analogy too far, it can be helpful to look at AIDS not in terms of shock, surprise, or disappointment (although those are appropriate early responses), but in terms of acceptance that awful things do happen in life. We have to learn to live as well as we can in any situation, in any set of circumstances—always remembering, however, that *acceptance* does not necessarily imply either *compliance* or *complacency*.

This is a very fine distinction—and a very important one. Too often we confuse acceptance with powerlessness, yet there is no necessary connection between the two. Just because you understand and accept the tragedy of AIDS does not mean that you are doomed to comply with its tragic course. Accepting that AIDS is a terrible thing, that it has altered our lives forever, that it may indeed claim your own life at some future point does not mean that you should simply give up and abandon yourself to wild living in order to facilitate the "inevitable."

Nor does it mean that you must become complacent, thinking that since this horrible thing is here, you may as well do your best to ignore it. That is yet another mode of denial, and will eventually bring you round, willy-nilly, to the sudden shock of re-awakening to the painful facts again and again.

I T took me many years and many visits to the therapist to accept that life was never going to return to "normal." I kept repeating to myself and to my friends that I just wished I could regain that old feeling of excitement about life—that unburdened feeling of enthusiasm that used to help me bounce out of bed in the morning, eager and hopeful, rather than awaken to the reality of a tough crisis that threatens to occupy life for a long time.

I have had to accept that it won't be that way ever again. There is simply no way to erase what has happened, or to forget the knowledge I have gained, or to escape the prospect of what is yet to come, whatever that may be.

Once I accepted that we are living life under the sword and that I will never feel exactly the way I once had, a curious thing happened. I began to cope with the crisis in a way I never had before. I began to feel quite justifiably angry— at the disease, at ignorance, at everything that wasn't being done. And with that acceptance and anger came a new spirit—not the same spirit of plain enthusiasm I once felt about life—but a new spirit that is just as eager and just as energetic about living life as it now is.

And so, reality can also be spectacular. To stop long enough to look, think, evaluate, and comprehend just what is and what is not real is a tool that leads to rich living. It enables us to make plans, to decide what the next step should be, to move ahead into life with determination and hope.

Chapter Six

SURRENDER

ACCEPTING reality is only one step in a long process of letting yourself move freely—even adventurously—into the future. But while one may freely banter about a phrase like "accepting reality" or letting yourself "surrender," most of us are hard pressed to understand what such concepts mean in concrete terms. What can a person actually *do* to accept and surrender? And what are the pitfalls along the way?

Accepting reality *can* lead to stagnation. One can simply give up, adopting a posture that, it would seem, is realistic in its confrontation with hopelessness. It can be very easy to tell oneself that okay, this is horrible, I'm not going to pretend this isn't happening, but I'm going to enjoy myself as long as I can.

This leads to a lifestyle of "living it up." Becoming fatalistic—thinking that whatever will be will be—is the greatest pitfall when one starts to adopt a realistic viewpoint about AIDS and about the changes the gay community is experiencing. It's an easy trap—you emerge from the darkness of denial, wake up and look around at the tragedy, and tell yourself that it's useless.

Accepting reality can also lead to severe depression—quite the opposite of living it up in the face of a grim fate. A

friend of mine endured several months of crushing, agoniz-
ing depression. He was so filled with the reality and hopelessness of AIDS facts that he had a tremendous struggle
on his hands every time he simply wanted to get up in the
morning. Overwhelmed by the regular display of statistics
in the newspaper and the nightly news, with its dreadful
hysterical reporting, he was kept in a fit of constant anxiety.

But every difficult challenge in life can include the germ
of tremendous, hopeful change as well. There *can* be a silver
lining in the cloud. Of course, it would be wrong, selfish,
and even uncompassionate to view AIDS—as some people
do—as an "important gift" or "lesson" from the "Universe." AIDS is not a gift of the universe. AIDS is not
something that was sent here to allow us to grow or to learn
important lessons in life.

Finding a silver lining in the cloud is difficult. Perhaps
the phrase "finding a silver lining" isn't very accurate, because it implies that there *is* a silver lining. What is really
meant here is that we can *create* a silver lining for ourselves
if we put our mind to it. We can give ourselves the chance
to view the tribulations of AIDS as a way to discover new
things about ourselves and as a way to forge new lifestyles.

The option always exists to sink into despair, realizing
that AIDS may indeed claim many of our friends and even
ourselves. The positive choice here is to accept AIDS for
what it is and to find the new ways we can live that are
satisfying and healthy.

But it's important to remember that *we* are giving these
meanings *to* the disease; they are not inherent in its actual-
ity. A lining is only one side of a garment, and we don't deny

that there is the outer fabric; the lining simply makes the garment more comfortable.

T HE intermediate step—between accepting the hard facts about AIDS and achieving a new understanding of life and its joys—is surrender.

Surrender is not, however, the same as giving away our options. Surrender is not a matter of yielding to fate. Surrender is more a matter of giving up the ability to hide from the facts. Surrender means acceptance *and* change. Surrender means that we must abandon the struggle—not the struggle against the disease in terms of helping others, living healthfully, working for education and funding—but abandoning the struggle to hide from the facts of AIDS.

This is a subtle distinction. So much of gay politics (and the liberal agenda in general) is articulated in terms of the "fight," the "battle" against oppressive forces. It is couched in militaristic terms, as if there were an "enemy" we would shoot down, destroy—and *overcome*.

But this kind of thinking is inherently negative. It defines the world in terms of oppositions—good vs. bad, right vs. wrong. Given such a definition, gay people cast themselves, then, in the role of victims, struggling valiantly against the evil forces which would oppress us.

Participating in that kind of thinking when it comes to AIDS merely perpetuates it, and that kind of thinking is futile, impotent.

Do not become a part of the drama. By fighting back,

we're perpetuating the cycle that defines the world in terms of me vs. you, them vs. us. All that can happen then are temporary victories and temporary setbacks, a constant, endless see-saw that does nothing but trade negativity for negativity.

There is a significant difference between political oppression and the oppression we feel because of AIDS. With political oppression, if one sees things as a struggle against the oppressors, at least there is someone against which to direct one's work. With AIDS, the object of our alarm is much more elusive. It is not just the virus and its attendant disease syndrome that worries us—though that by itself would surely be enough. We also worry about the problems of our friends and lovers, of our community, of this dreadful black cloud hanging over our heads. It is the fact of being catapulted—without choice—into a sudden culture of illness that weighs heavily on our mind. To get beyond that is the difficult task of surrender.

S URRENDER means that we step beyond the regular definitions of the "struggle." It's rather like watching a play or an opera. Think about yourself on stage, deciding that no, you're no longer interested in playing out the drama. You step off stage and observe the action from the wings, or from the audience. Watch all the players act out their parts. You tell yourself that you're really not very interested in *that* story; you'd rather have a different story altogether. As a matter of fact, you'd rather not have any story at all. You'd rather have the opera end so that you can attend to the things that are at hand. Whether it's changing your eating habits, exercising, meditating, quitting smoking, donating time and money to care for the dying, writing letters to the editor . . . whatever you need to do *outside* the drama, you need to do now!

Surrender means that you've decided that you're going to put aside the roles, negative thoughts, and habits you've been accumulating. You're not going to see AIDS as anything other than what it is. You're not going to be haunted by the past. You're not going to wake up every morning and wonder just why bother getting out of bed.

You're going to surrender to the reality of whatever comes next. You're going to do what you can do today, this moment. You're going to understand that you don't know what comes next, and that perhaps you only vaguely know what happened before. You're going to understand that all you can really know is the present moment. And you're going to know that your task is right here, right now.

This might seem to be a solipsism, as if each individual can know only what is happening in terms of himself or herself. It might also seem to be some kind of smarmy mumbo-jumbo that relieves you of your responsibility to others.

But it is neither a solipsism nor mumbo-jumbo. It is an attitude and a choice. In many ways, surrender is allowing yourself to develop the ability to shrug your shoulders. So what if things used to seem more fun? So what if the baths and sex clubs used to be open? So what if it's harder to get up in the morning and go on with your life? So what if things aren't the way they used to be?

Oh, it's easy to be flippant about the very real concerns that bother us day after day. The problem for many people is the constant nagging in the back of our minds—we find that the inner dialogue just won't stop, that the small inner voice continues its harangue: . . . *what happened? . . . will it ever end? . . . will I get sick and die? . . . will my friends? . . . I miss the old days . . . it was so wonderful . . .*

The act of shrugging your shoulders to such inner worries is the act of surrender, of making a conscious choice not to dwell in the land of woes. The friend of mine who had suffered so much with depression told me that he finally had to get hold of himself and *force* himself to think of other things, to worry about something else, to acknowledge that of course he was very concerned—and would remain so—but that fretting over it day and night was ruining his life. He formed a new habit. Whenever he would find the inner voice going on and on with worry, he would first picture a cassette recorder, the tape playing on endlessly. Then he imagined that he was pushing the stop button. Then he imagined that he put some nice music on, jazz or classical. Then he imagined that he turned away from the cassette player and looked out the window at a forest, or a field of wildflowers, or the beach.

This might sound corny, but the point is that we do have control over what we think. We can make conscious decisions about our inner dialogue and worries, just as we can choose what to say, where to have lunch, when to go to bed. Surrendering to reality involves breaking habits that keep us stuck in denial or anxiety. Surrendering means letting go, and what we let go of is denial, anxiety, and the *habits* that reinforce negativity.

Chapter Seven

TRANSFORMATION

THERE was a time when we used to go on and off diets, stop and start smoking, attend the gym and then give it up, become vegetarians for a week and then return to carnivorous ways. Health fads came and went with regularity, and we gave them little more thought than we would deciding which program to watch on television.

Now the stakes are too high for fads. Now we accept that we don't want to take chances with improper diet, cigarettes, liquor, lack of exercise, no peace of mind. It's just not worth it. We're moving toward a new kind of fitness, one that embraces the classic ideals of soundness, peacefulness—inner and outer serenity.

We've learned about good nutrition, proper aerobic and anaerobic exercise, meditative rest, safe sex, and the value of love and caring for one another. We've learned how to support one another through terrible crises, through panics, diagnoses, and the omnipresent dark cloud over our heads.

It hasn't been easy, and it will never be easy. We have had—and are continuing to have—to learn skills and adaptive behaviors that are nothing like anything we ever expected to encounter. That struggle is plainly difficult, as if life has forced us to take a sharp detour that we would rather not have had to take.

But by yielding to life—by surrendering to a reality that is teaching us that things are not always easy, that life can dish out some tough times—we gain the ability to become the healthiest we can. Awakening to the facts, remembering what is important to us, accepting reality and eschewing escapism, surrendering to the flow of life and letting go of fear —these are the elements that allow transformation to occur.

This transformation is both physical and mental. The mental anguish and anxiety that we experience on a daily basis are so stressing that they often lead to a physical malaise: lethargy, lack of enthusiasm, feeling grouchy and frustrated, poor sleep, poor nutrition, and escapism.

Often, this malaise seems overwhelming, quite beyond anything we feel we have the strength to adapt to. When this feeling of malaise, this lousy mood, overtakes us, that's the critical time to retreat not to fantasy, but to reality. We have to sit down and have a talk with ourselves, remind ourselves that of course this isn't easy, but we have to do the best we can. Struggling to overcome depression, stress, and malaise is in itself a very courageous and positive act, and through it we are strengthened.

S OME of the changes we are experiencing have been forced on us—closure of bathhouses, favorite bars, and the departure of friends. The very real fear of AIDS has forced safe sex into practice and stimulated worries about just how well we are living, how healthfully we're leading our lives.

But much of the transformation is left for us to decide, and this is perhaps the toughest part of all. For how many times have each of us sat and wondered just what it is that we can do about the AIDS crisis in general, about our own health specifically, about the health of our friends and community? We read the papers, we hear stories from friends, we wonder: Is there a way to beat this thing? Is there something that each individual can do to stay well? To avoid illness? To survive the epidemic? To help others survive?

Deciding what to do about these things—and how to proceed, which means breaking old habits and establishing new ones, changing thought patterns and attitudes, setting up new relationships with our bodies for optimum health, researching the constantly changing news about treatment —is a critical and difficult challenge.

Recommendations from medical authorities are sometimes conflicting, or, at the very least, require actions about which we still feel unsure. We want to wait for the perfect solution, a better medicine, more evidence, a sudden breakthrough, a near-cure—all thoughts that come to us so easily when we're fearful or uncertain about facing new action, new habits, changes.

So we sit and frustrate our own transformation process, failing to make the crucial changes that might make the difference. But what are those crucial changes? Well, the answer is complex. Finding the answer to that question means finding a great deal of information and applying it to one's own life. That is difficult and demanding. We have to become our own medical experts. We have to read as much as we can, study the data that's available—both from the medical establishment and from the "fringes."

But this approach doesn't necessarily feel comfortable to us. In this country there is a strong tradition that places a great deal of faith in medical doctors—or in any kind of authority for that matter. We have been taught to believe—as so many television commercials state—that "doctors know best," as if medical authorities have all the answers and we, as individuals, have none. We have come to believe that we don't really have any control over our own health, at least not insofar as fighting serious disease is concerned. We've learned through experience that if you get very sick, you go to the doctor and get a pill or shot.

Many people are now questioning this blind faith in traditional authorities. Many people are questioning blind faith in *anyone*, including doctors, alternative health practitioners, faith healers, nutritionists. Many people are coming to believe that the individual can know what is best by educating himself as thoroughly as possible, then incorporating his intuitive feelings into the decisions he makes about health.

This questioning is not just another crazy fringe movement suggesting that individuals are somehow imbued with the natural ability to understand the complex machinery of the human body better than physicians. This skepticism is part of an overall movement suggesting that we need not sit idly by as if we did not have the power or learning ability to make good, informed decisions. It is possible to acquire a great deal of knowledge about health and about AIDS. It is possible to take that information and make sense of it in your own life. It is possible to become skeptical without debunking the entire medical establishment. It is possible to learn from alternative health practitioners without becoming a sappy goofball who hugs trees. It is possible to take much more responsibility for your own life and to realize that your decisions—and the habits you form because of them—can influence the person you are. We are not passive creatures who must sit "waiting for Godot." We can do something every day that expands our knowledge and reinforces our new habits, helping ourselves move along the path of transformation.

A T the very heart of transformation is the actual physical condition of your body—in short, what kind of health you're in. It isn't possible to choose the best way to transform yourself into the healthiest person you can be until you know where you stand right now. But a great many people fear that knowledge, because it can be a tremendous stress just by itself.

Medical experts tell us that if one is infected with the human immunodeficiency virus (HIV), then one is at greater risk of developing AIDS or ARC as more time goes by. It is believed that the AIDS virus wreaks havoc on the immune system as time passes, leaving the body open for infection. Symptoms begin to appear. The results of long-term, untreated HIV infection are very serious.

Yet doctors still have little to offer beyond further blood

tests, immunologic profiles, and treatment by some very useful but imperfect drugs, which we hesitate to use. Holistic health practitioners offer a variety of approaches, probably more than any one individual can research, let alone assimilate. And there exist, now, a number of "alternative" treatments that individuals can use to treat themselves or experimental drug trials that individuals can enter.

It is good to be aware that "alternative" is not synonymous with "fake." Alternative treatment means exactly that—it is treatment that is an alternative to standard medical practice. And it is good to be aware that "experimental" is not synonymous with "dangerous." Some experimental drug trials may be risky to be sure—but they may also give you a head start on a cure.

The thing to do about your fears, depression, anxiety, confusion, and health condition (whether simply worried, HIV infected, or have ARC or AIDS), is to become your own best health expert. Do not shy away from confronting reality. Do not avoid the news. Research all the news reports, the many available books, the many newsletters describing alternative treatments or experimental drugs. Consider the experiences and opinions of others who have tried different approaches. Then, take all this information and find a balanced approach that suits your particular situation—your health needs, your lifestyle. Listen to your own heart—to that inner voice that is very discerning—and follow its lead, provided, of course, that its lead is not along a path of denial or fear. Fear and denial must be eschewed, for they cripple transformation.

The approach that many people now follow is, first, to discover their status as antibody positive or negative. If positive, they have gone on to have complete medical workups done—especially T-cell counts—in order to determine the actual condition of their general health and specifically of their immune systems. If, in fact, their medical tests show that their immune systems are suffering as a result of HIV infection, they begin immediate treatment with an anti-viral—either one of the approved anti-viral drugs or one (or more) of the alternative or experimental anti-virals. The scope of options available is variable and changes with time. (For a long time, AZT was the only "approved" anti-viral, but then came ddI on the parallel track, and a number of potential anti-virals available through clinical trials.)

Next, they examine their lives closely, to see to what extent they are doing their best to stay well. The easiest thing to do, of course, is simply to "live better" with proper nutrition, exercise, and rest. They forswear proven poisons like liquor, tobacco, recreational drugs, and food that is nutritionally bankrupt. They adopt a mixed routine of exercise that includes aerobic exercise for fitness, endurance, and strength (swimming, calisthenics, aerobics classes, running, light weightlifting, bicycling) and some other activity for balance and centering (yoga, stretching, bodywork).

And then they have focussed on that part of life that we so often overlook, the spiritual, doing things that feed the spirit like meditation, relaxation exercises, prayer, walking in nature, viewing art, listening to music, and a variety of spiritual techniques.

They have completely altered their outlook on sexual expression, seeking close friends or lovers who are nurturing and supportive, who cooperate willingly and cheerfully in safe sex only.

And they have begun to live with a sense of hope, knowing that a cure may be found, that *maintaining* healthful practices and anti-viral therapy is the best approach.

Of course many people refuse to begin their transformation, or they dabble, doing a little meditation now and then, starting an exercise program for a while, *thinking* about AZT, and so on. Refusing to begin your transformation is something along the lines of the ostrich burying its head in the sand. But it's far more dangerous than that, because allowing a suppressed immune system to remain untreated will become deadly. Refusing to gather all the information needed for transformation is denial. Refusing to act on that information if and when it is gathered is foolish. AIDS infection is not something to ignore.

A friend of mine refused for many years to take the test for antibodies to the AIDS virus. He fussed and worried, unwilling to face the fact that he might be infected. When he finally began to feel very tired on a daily basis, he went and had the test done. Discovering that he was indeed infected, he went to his doctor and requested a full workup, including the blood panels that would show the condition of his immune system, specifically the T-cell count. It turned out that his immune system had been seriously damaged by the AIDS infection, to the point that he was well within the "danger zone." Several of his friends tried to educate him about the treatment options available, but he just laughed and said, "You've got to be kidding." Try as we might, we couldn't convince him that he was in a serious position, but yet lucky enough to be relatively symptom free—which is the best time to intervene with treatment.

He wouldn't hear of it, and after several months of seemingly good health (which he misinterpreted to mean that he was "fine"), he developed pneumocystis pneumonia and subsequently a number of other serious infections.

Other friends have taken a different path. Upon discovering that they were infected with the AIDS virus and that their immune systems were suppressed to one degree or another, they embarked upon a series of transformations that weren't especially easy, but were accomplished nevertheless. Nearly all of these friends immediately began antiviral therapy, using standard, alternative, and/or experimental therapies for their HIV infection. And they worked to adopt the healthiest lifestyle they could—including adequate rest, excellent nutrition, exercise, and some form of meditative work.

Of course there are no guarantees, because every human body is different, every physical constitution highly individual. But you've got to give yourself a fighting chance. The best treatment/health regimen can't guarantee its outcome, but not to try is certainly weak of spirit and medically proven to be dangerous. My friend who refused to consider treatment—after bothering to take the test and find out how poorly his immune system was functioning—acted foolishly by refusing to complete the process of transformation. He got only halfway there, by learning the condition of his health. But he couldn't face, for whatever reasons, the pros-

pect of medical treatment and lifestyle changes, thereby
aborting the chances he might have created for himself
through early intervention. He just never gave himself a
fighting chance.

There is no one, sanctioned approach, but there is one
undeniable truth: Transformation is necessary. The things
that make up "transformation" are variable. But gone is the
day when people went about their lives without knowing
their immune status, when they refused to begin treatment
because of uncertainty. Now is the day to "take the bull by
the horns" and take action.

By taking action in a real, physical way, an emotional
transformation occurs, creating an overall transformation
that is complete and that lets us sleep at night. Until we do
everything that we can do, the stress of knowing that we are
letting ourselves down will remain a strong and overwhelming part of life. You can't examine the stress; you have to
examine what you are *doing* about the stress. You can't examine the panic; you have to struggle against it. You can't
sit and wonder what your medical status is; you have to find
out. You can't accept that you are helpless to cope with infection; you have to discover what can be done and then do
it. You *can* transform your health into the best it can be,
within the limits of your circumstances, no matter what
doubts may haunt you.

Once you've decided on a plan, the next thing to do is to
solicit support for your program—support from friends,
family, your lover. Tell them that you've decided to do such-
and-such in order to maximize good health, and tell them

what they can do to help you—to keep an open mind, to give you the freedom to select new habits and implement them.

Get your doctor's support, too. Ideally, you'll have worked out your "good health plan" with your doctor's advice, but failing that, let him or her know what you're doing and ask for support—in terms of being available to answer questions, being willing to order any lab tests necessary to monitor your progress, promising to call you with any new information. If your doctor isn't supportive, then change doctors. Ask friends who are taking responsibility for their health who their doctors are.

Once you've done all these things and are well along your path of seeking good health, any sense of helplessness should dissipate. Of course, from time to time everyone has moments of despair and anxiety. But as long as you know that you're doing everything that you can to maximize your health, those fears can't overwhelm you. You'll be moving on with a renewed sense of vitality and hopefulness.

Chapter Eight

HOPE

THE good feeling of hope is something that many of us have lost. If you think you're doomed, then you can't have hope. Hope exists in the belief that you can live, that you *want* to live, that you'll do anything you can to keep on living.

Before going any further, let me state a fact. The fact about AIDS and the gay community is this: We are not doomed.

If we give up, if we concede to fear and hopelessness, then yes, we're doomed. But if we insist on living—on surviving—and if we do everything we can do to ensure that we will survive (lifestyle changes, healthy living, and medical and alternative treatments), then *we are not doomed*.

Many historians point out that the greatest victory the Nazis ever had was that of convincing the Jews that they were doomed. Without the hopelessness of that belief in a doomed future, the Jews could never have been forced into submission. It was the wholesale concession to a doomed future that allowed the Nazis to carry out their hideous plan with such alarming ease.

While there may or may not be an overarching and conscious attempt to persuade the gay community that it is doomed by the spectre of AIDS, the fact remains that such a notion is unfortunately widespread. This doom-and-gloom is in large part a product of the manner in which the media report the findings of scientists and epidemiologists. We tend, perhaps too often, to lay blame for public panic at the doors of science and epidemiology—yet they have their very good and productive role. The role of epidemiological statistics is worthwhile, yet the glee with which the media extract horror stories from those *ever-changing* statistics is a travesty. It is true that our society's blatant homophobia is well served by this notion of doom, and that by itself is enough to taint news reportage with the underlying presumption that death is surely the only thing that awaits the gay community today.

The gay community must not accept such thinking. That we have allowed this ideology of doom to paralyze us with fear is shocking, and all the more so because rebellion against prevailing thought has always been what the gay community is all about. If "they" tell us that we're doomed, ought we not to rebel against that notion with a liberal dose of skepticism and bravado?

Of course, there is good reason for people to have abandoned hope and cowered under the spectre of AIDS. It has been a terrible, terrible tragedy, an ugly, hideous mess of the worst proportions. Not only is it an awful disease to endure, but our society has often turned on people with AIDS in a grim and merciless way. It has proven to be too much for us to assimilate, and the overwhelming nature of the epidemic has robbed us of hope and has often created this sense of doom.

HOPE

For a very long time I lived without hope. Years of reading the newspapers had eroded my hope to such a point that I truly believed everything was hopeless—life, work, relationships, health, the possibility of a cure. Day after day I would read of the epidemiologic forecasts, would watch the death toll mount, would hear the "grim" reports that a cure or a vaccine was years away—and over time, these reports took their toll on my attitude. My hopefulness simply dried up. I began to suffer from a common form of AIDS hysteria—fatigue and hypochondria. I became angry and belligerent, hostile to my co-workers, my lover, family, and friends. If one's hope is obscured, the world is a very ugly place—there is simply nothing worth living for.

The shadow of AIDS casts a gloomy spell over any hope. It can even obscure hope completely, robbing the future of any pleasure, as if nothing that will happen next can bring even the faintest moment of relief from the suffering of friends, from the onward march of the disease, from the continuing and crippling fear. With the mounting statistics and the hysterical news reports, one can lose all perspective, all sense that perhaps, someday, we'll have a day when AIDS will be gone, when the fear will have passed, when we can get on with our lives without the doomed mood we have come to know so well.

My own hopelessness eventually dissipated, and I regained a hopeful outlook on life and the future. But before I tell that story, the subject of hope should be defined.

HOPE is a thought, feeling, or emotion that exists naturally. Hope is as human as breathing. Hope is simply to want something when there exists the expectation or possibility of fulfillment. One can hope that the future will be pleasant because in one's experience the future has often turned out to be so. One can also hope that the future will get better, because one knows that things are being done to assure that it will be so. One can not hope that the future will include the resurrection of a favorite family pet that has long since died, because, of course, there is no reasonable expectation that such a thing can come to pass. That would fall under the definition of a wish, or perhaps faith.

Hope is something that is directed towards an object or a goal. We all have "hopes for the future," when we'll travel or own a home or be successful in our careers. In our mind's eye we maintain a vague vision of how things will be in the future, of all the things we will accomplish and enjoy.

Some hopes are more immediate than others. I hope to visit my mother next month, and I also hope to spend a year in a cabin in the woods some day. I hope my car doesn't break down in heavy traffic when I drive downtown this morning, and I also hope that I will go to Mexico next spring. All of these little hopes create a mixture of optimism and good feelings about the future—the feeling that there's something to which to look forward.

Hope, then, is something that exists from the earliest moment in our lives.

THAT hope can be obscured—because the expected outcome seems distant, impossible, or because everyone around us is telling us to abandon all hope—is a very real danger, and when it comes to the AIDS crisis, the fact that hope is obscured by our failing expectations is very serious. It's very serious because this is a time when we can least afford to give up hope. Hope is the great motivator. Without hope, we tend to become despondent, languishing in inaction, fretting in indecision. With the AIDS crisis, we need to be active and decisive more than ever. AIDS demands nothing but the very best from us, the most decisive action, the clearest thinking, the greatest hopefulness.

But what is there to be hopeful about? Aren't the statistics and predictions absolutely dreadful? Aren't we given to understand that unless there's some medical breakthrough, thousands upon thousands are doomed to die of AIDS?

Well, the answers to these questions are not as easy as they might seem. The statistics and predictions are indeed dreadful, but they are precisely that—predictions. What is predicted is not necessarily going to happen, though, unless things change, those predictions will probably prove to be as accurate as they have been up until now.

But the key phrase here—and it's the one that gives us hope—is "unless things change." Things can change; things do change. In fact, things already are changing. The advent of the drug AZT has changed the medical treatment of AIDS and ARC in a very major, very positive way, and while it is by no means a cure, it is one great step in the direction of effective long-term treatment of the disease. Not too long ago, there was no such medicine available.

The presence and availability of other medicines and substances to treat AIDS, ARC, and HIV infection is evolving rapidly. Already there are many experimental treatments from which to choose, and as time goes by, there will undoubtedly be many more. And as people treat themselves with these alternatives, or take AZT and live as healthfully as they can, the drug companies and medical researchers are refining existing medicines, testing new ones, experimenting with others, researching new chemical formulae and substances. There is something to be hopeful about.

As people realize that there is hope, and as they work toward good health by taking steps to improve their health, and, if they choose to, treat themselves with unapproved medications so that they can "hang on" (to put it bluntly), then there is even more to be hopeful about. Because what can happen is this—people who are infected can slow down their progression toward illness, perhaps halt it, long enough to wait for the good outcome we all hope for—a cure or a good, effective treatment.

For this reason—that there are things we each can do, and more things are approaching—we can hope. This *is* something new, however, because it has only been recently that we have had any treatment options whatsoever.

That one fact is changing everything for the more hopeful. What once was a fairly bleak situation is no longer hopeless.

WAKING up to this fact is a problem, because the feeling of doom is terribly widespread. And while this is not going to be an easy crisis to surmount, and many more of our friends will undoubtedly pass away, it is important that each of us take some action as soon as possible to foster hope, to persuade ourselves to get busy to get well (or stay well).

If one lives without hope, sooner or later one comes to the old "existential crisis," where one either does oneself in or finds some reason to go on. This sounds extreme when laid out so plainly on paper, but I know that I lived through it—more than once—and I know that most of my friends have struggled with it as well. You lay there in bed one day and realize that you just can't go on with things the way they are. It's just not worth it. You have the strongest feeling that *something* has got to change.

What has to change—I finally realized in my own life—is both thinking and behavior. It might sound simplistic, but that's what hope can do for you. It is simple. It's a matter of focussing your mind on something *good* and *positive* in the future, such as the day they announce an effective treatment or cure for AIDS, and in the meantime taking the necessary steps to be sure that you'll see that day.

If you're not worried about surviving, because you know that you're not infected with AIDS, and you're absolutely resolved to remain that way through healthy living with safe sex only, then you can still take action in hope by volunteering to help out answering phones at a crisis center, or participating in fundraisers, or contributing to AIDS research, or volunteering to care for people with AIDS by becoming a "buddy" through one of the many AIDS support service organizations.

But it's important to do *something*, to take some action.

The way into hope is the way that involves work, action, doing things. Action is stimulated by hope, and hope produces action. I think that many people have actually been *afraid* of hope, because hope leads to action, and action can mean changing lifestyles, seeking medical or experimental treatments, and it can pose other "disruptions" to life. Rather than face the realities that such action implies, it is easier to abandon the possibility of hope. Passive despair has become comfortable. People have accepted passivity as the *only* approach to the AIDS crisis—the idea that we'll "just wait and see." Well, we've waited, and we've seen, and there's no good that comes of that.

O NCE we take action, our mental processes work to clear away illusions and misinformation, and in the doing we suddenly find that we haven't got time for fear or depression or anxiety or any of the unproductive emotions. There's just too much to be done to waste time fretting.

What got me going again was a sudden moment of doubt. One day, while talking to a friend who was very skeptical about everything that was being reported about AIDS, I began to share his skepticism. I wondered if perhaps the grim forecasts might be wrong. Perhaps there might be a cure in the very near future.

This moment of skeptical doubt remained foremost in my mind for several days. I realized that it had been only a very short while back—in 1983—that they'd discovered the AIDS virus. I remembered that up until that point there had been mere speculation, one wild theory after another. All kinds of wacky theories were being put forth about AIDS—from the notion that poppers caused AIDS to the crazy idea that it was some sort of germ warfare.

Well, I realized, we've come quite a distance in a few years. We're now dealing in hard, scientific fact, in laboratory evidence, in the measurable, workable world of microscopes and biochemistry. Promising experimental drugs have been developed in astonishingly short periods of time, and who's to know how quickly the next breakthrough will come?

In one sudden, spectacular moment, I envisioned a day in the future—after we had all been into our doctors' offices for our treatments—when I would look back on this time of my life and think about "those dark times in my early thirties when I wasn't really so sure I was going to make it."

It was this that altered my attitude, that fostered a new mood of hope. After envisioning that day in the future, everything else seemed much easier. The idea of changing my lifestyle to include the healthiest habits I could didn't seem any great constraint. To exercise regularly, to eliminate foods that aren't nutritious, to add a daily meditation for relaxation into my schedule, to look into vitamins or other supplements that might help boost immunity, to educate myself about the experimental treatments that are available should they be called for—what are these other than plain, simple tasks? With this good feeling of hope, they seemed the easiest things in the world to do.

Rather than fret about the hopelessness of AIDS, I decided to focus on the possibility of a cure. And I began to question what might be hindering progress in that direction. If I could identify the factors that slow the progress toward a cure, then I could determine what I could do—in real life, not just in attitude—to help. I tried fundraising, volunteering, writing letters to legislators and to the media, and writing books to help people. And once I started to do these things, the hopelessness dissipated and I felt a great resurgence of hopefulness, of optimism, of knowing that something *could* be done about AIDS—that something *was* being done.

Creating a new mood of hope was the same pathway as eliminating the terror of AIDS. Where I had had to work on eliminating fear by forming new physical habits, I now had to work on eliminating hopelessness by doing something that would lead to the outcome we all want—an end to the AIDS crisis.

The secret to creating and maintaining hope is to know that hope leads to action. When you hope that you'll have a new car next year, you don't expect the new car to materialize in front of you some morning. Instead, you take some action, you make some plans—you study your budget so that you can save enough money for a down payment; perhaps you take a sack lunch to the office for six months to save that money. You visit auto dealerships on weekends and talk to friends, so that you can gather all the information you'll need to make your choice.

Finding hope during the AIDS crisis is precisely the same thing. You recognize your hopeful goals—to survive, to help your friends survive, to give comfort to those who won't, to help alleviate fear, to help educate the public so that the disease is prevented, and to help the progress toward a cure.

Once you've listed your hopeful goals you can outline your plan about what you're going to do to reach them—starting with learning everything about the state of your own health so that you can adopt a treatment and healthy living plan, then moving on to do something for the community and to help overcome the crisis: to volunteer to answer phones, to hand out pamphlets, to donate money, to organize and participate in fundraisers, become involved in free "guerilla clinics," participate in public protests, whatever—and then you do it.

And in the doing, you discover that yes, your world has changed, that indeed life is not what you had planned, but that, in renewed hope, in peace of mind and good spirits, you have achieved an inner balance—serenity.

AFTERWORD

I DIDN'T originally intend to write the kind of book that contains a resource directory, annotated bibliography, or that mentions specific treatment substances. My original intent was to write a series of essays that would simply reflect the experience that so many of us are enduring, so that in the reading, people could identify with my experience and find comfort.

But as the book evolved, and as I moved further into the chapters on transformation and hope, I realized that a collection of essays on the general experience of AIDS in the gay community wasn't enough. Too many of my friends were ignoring their own health in an effort to "wait and see" what the researchers were coming up with that it became obvious that something more was needed in the way of a resource that would stimulate and inspire people to *do* something about AIDS.

Rather than pleasant dinner table conversations about movies and weekend plans, I noticed that people were constantly discussing AIDS in dismal terms of hopelessness— as if we were all cowering under the table, waiting for the axe to fall, refusing to take any action. This made me angry.

But examining my own experience—which resulted in the first two-thirds of this book—taught me that we have been lulled into a dangerous passivity, that our fear has overwhelmed our common sense, that the reason we fail to motivate ourselves into action is because we have been fooled into believing that there is no action that is worthwhile.

This is why I let the book evolve into something more than a collection of essays. I certainly don't want to preach; I have neither the credentials nor the chutzpah for that. And I certainly don't assert that I know a step-by-step program that will assure long life and happiness. But I do know the road, with all its twists, turns, and false starts. Perhaps this book can act as a map.

—PAUL REED
October 1987
San Francisco

POSTSCRIPT

SINCE writing this book in 1986/1987, I could have added a new chapter and called it "Acceptance." Of all the lessons I have had to learn in recent years, it has been acceptance that is the most important—to accept life, pain, turmoil, grief, and loss. And in the heart of accepting lies peace—not happiness, but peace.

In the past three years I have faced my own HIV infection and lost my lover, to whom this book is dedicated, to AIDS. It has been a hard thing to live amidst such pain and still maintain a health regimen, still struggle against HIV infection, still maintain some degree of hope. Yes, as my lover grew sicker and as I faced my own health risks in declining T-cells, I found it increasingly difficult to continue a health regimen. Yet I *have* done so, using a variety of treatment approaches, adjusting, monitoring, changing, and watching. And when the emotional pain reached a howling pitch, I increased my anti-stress efforts—long walks, meditation, journal work, relaxation exercises, and so on. For in the midst of such distractingly high emotions, these are the only real tools we have.

It has been the hardest challenge of my life and the greatest lesson to learn that even when I had done *everything I could*, I might still remain in anguish, simply because the burden was so heavy, the issues so deep, the loss so encompassing. But we must accept it and stick with it. Even in our darkest moments, by remaining faithful to our health regimens, by accepting the support of loving friends, by reminding ourselves that we're in the middle of a dreadful epidemic, and by reaching for the future, we can help reduce the physical and emotional effects of all this stress. We can't make everything all right; we can't necessarily feel "good" or "normal;" but we *can* keep at it, working *towards* health, *towards* acceptance, *towards* peace. It is this process that is life.

But beyond my own life and concerns, it has been heartening to see how strongly the community has pulled together as the epidemic worsens. We are doing many things—from the compassion of hospice programs to the angry demonstrations of ACT-UP—and there has been a real resurgence in the sense of our *community*, that we are all in this together, that we *can* make a difference, and that, perhaps, we can find an effective therapy and convert HIV infection into a manageable chronic condition.

But it has also been maddening to watch the snail's pace at which treatment research has moved, to see with dismay that national leadership is still lacking, to witness the loss of more friends and lovers who might have been spared had research been supported and rushed—in short, if AIDS had been treated like the emergency that it is. Why, after a decade of the epidemic, it is still regarded as something on the fringes instead of the devastating global catastrophe that it is, is mystifying at best, horrifying at worst. The only true serenity we're going to achieve is when we have raised enough of a ruckus to cure this epidemic. We must all try to live to see that day.

—PAUL REED
May 1990
San Francisco

RESOURCES

FINDING a way through this epidemic requires a great deal of personal effort and education. This section lists some books, newsletters, and organizations that are very helpful in dealing with the sorts of questions and problems that living with the AIDS crisis brings up. There are considerably more resources available that can be of enormous help in coping with AIDS, illness, stress, good health, and loss, but listed here are only those that have been the most helpful to me. Most of the books listed here contain resource directories or bibliographies of their own, and looking through them is an excellent way to search out further information.

BOOKS AND NEWSLETTERS (in alphabetical order by title):

Afterlife, by Paul Monette (New York, NY: Crown Publishers, 1990). A stirring look at the lives of surviving partners—AIDS "widowers"—this novel by the author of the excellent memoir *Borrowed Time* is useful not only as a good novel, but as a way of helping one through grief, something that all of us must deal with as the multiple losses mount.

Ultimately a love story, *Afterlife* shows that life *does* go on, sometimes difficult, sometimes mystifying, sometimes joyous. Fiction can touch us in ways that nonfiction, visual, and interpersonal communications can't, and *Afterlife* is worthwhile for this reason. Monette is a bit gloomy about the prospects of HIV-infected people, but it is just one expression of a dark reality that we all must consider if we're to confront our illness—and eventual mortality as well.

AIDS: A Self-Care Manual, by Betty Clare Moffatt, *et al.* (Los Angeles, CA: IBS Press, 1987). Divided according to subjects—social, medical, treatment, prevention, etc.—this book is a standard tool in helping sort your way through your own treatment plan and health regimen. It is very helpful in sorting out the various aspects of one's life and how to deal with them in a healthy way in the context of fighting HIV disease.

AIDS and Its Metaphors, by Susan Sontag (New York, NY: Farrar, Straus & Giroux, 1989). This brief volume extends Sontag's earlier *Illness as Metaphor* to analyze the ramifications of AIDS. Her basic message is that we tend to invest events such as an epidemic with "meanings" far beyond what little may be factually implied and that often these meanings cause serious problems—such as guilt, injustice, discrimination, even needless worry. Very helpful is her relentless deconstruction of myths about AIDS—its being God's punishment for sin or the result of psychological predispositions, for example. She doesn't say that AIDS is without meaning, but she does show that many aspects of our thinking about AIDS are related historically to cultural and social themes that continue to repeat themselves regardless of differing circumstances and differing eras. To her credit, Sontag does not offer her own or "better" meanings. Rather she allows that people may find their own meanings, though within the context of awareness of historical trends with regard to illness, plague, and so on. The book, then, is wonderfully liberating to read, because it helps in identifying areas of misguided thinking.

AIDS Treatment News, published biweekly by John S. James, P.O. Box 411256, San Francisco, CA 94141; phone (415) 255–0588. This biweekly newsletter is perhaps the best source of information on alternative and experimental treatments for AIDS, ARC, and HIV infection. It is also a critical resource for understanding the entire problem of treatment research. It is available by subscription, and back issues are available in paperback book form.

AIDS/HIV Experimental Treatment Directory, published by AmFAR (American Foundation for AIDS Research), 1515 Broadway, New York, NY 10036-8901; phone (212) 719-0033 (credit card orders only). This quarterly directory, available for $30 a year (free to people with AIDS or ARC), reports on all compounds being tested for AIDS treatment, with a focus on the status of all the clinical trials that are going on. Though highly technical, this is also the most complete "overview" of AIDS treatment research; by maintaining a thorough understanding of everything going on in AIDS research, patients are empowered with knowledge that can be an important component of planning personal treatment strategies.

Anatomy of an Illness as Perceived by the Patient, by Norman
Cousins (New York, NY: W. W. Norton Co., 1979). As inspiring as it is informative, this is perhaps the most well-
known and most convincing book about the importance of
a positive attitude in achieving and maintaining good
health. The author was stricken with a terrifying disease,
but through determination and the application of laughter,
he was able to heal himself and recover. While AIDS, ARC,
and HIV infection are indeed different, Norman Cousins's
story is a good introduction to some of the basic tenets
within the holistic health and wellness movement.

And the Band Played On, by Randy Shilts (New York, NY:
St. Martin's Press, 1987). Controversial and infuriating in
what it shows about this country's approach to AIDS, this
book is the most definitive history of the AIDS epidemic.
Many people disagree with the passionate narrative, but it
serves a purpose in bringing home the alarming nature of
the AIDS epidemic and the way in which it has been so
often sidestepped by government and industry.

BETA (Bulletin of Experimental Treatments for AIDS), published by the San Francisco AIDS Foundation, P.O. Box
6182, San Francisco, CA 94101; phone (415) 863–AIDS.
BETA offers in-depth, monthly reports, in layman's terms,
on anti-virals and other treatment substances. One of its
strong points for people in the Northern California area is
its directory to ongoing clinical trials in the region.

Bibliography of AIDS-Related Books, compiled by Sasha Alyson (Boston, MA: Alyson Publications, 1989). Put together

as a service to the bookselling industry, this bibliography lists nearly 200 books about AIDS and includes an evaluation of the value of each. This little bibliography can serve as a list of available books and guide you to those that are worthwhile. The bibliography is available by sending a 6″×9″ or larger envelope with two first-class stamps to Alyson Publications, 40 Plympton Street, Boston, MA 02118, with a note requesting the bibliography.

The Courage to Grieve, by Judy Tatelbaum (New York, NY: Harper & Row, 1980). Part of the process of maintaining personal balance and coping with stress is to process our grief consciously and well. With the multiple losses that come with an epidemic, we're often overwhelmed by grief, yet sometimes we may not even know that we're grieving. This book is a wonderful tool in bringing grief to the level of clear awareness, allowing us to understand our feelings, express them appropriately, and move on with our lives.

Face to Face: A Guide to AIDS Counseling, edited by James W. Dilley, Cheri Pies, and Michael Helquist (San Francisco, CA: The AIDS Health Project, University of California, San Francisco, 1989). Intended primarily for mental health professionals—counselors, psychiatrists, psychologists, social workers—and other AIDS caregivers, this book can be enormously comforting in its wealth of information. The book covers a wide range of issues, from antibody testing to neurological complications in AIDS. Its plain language is a blessing—no heavy academic jargon here—and its advice to therapists can be easily personalized by patients, friends, and families.

How To Persuade Your Lover To Use a Condom . . . And Why You Should, by Patti Breitman, Kim Knutson, and Paul Reed (Sacramento, CA: Prima Publishing, distributed by St. Martin's Press, New York, 1987). I wrote this book with my co-authors because we were angry at the way everyone was screaming "use a condom" without giving the down-to-earth, plain-talking advice people need in order to get into the habit of using condoms. We deliberately maintained a sex-positive, optimistic tone, yet presented forceful arguments anyone can use. If you're having trouble making the change to safe sex only, this book might help.

PI Perspective, published tri-annually by Project Inform, 347 Dolores Street, Suite 301, San Francisco, CA 94110; phone (415) 558-9051; toll-free (800) 334-7422 (within California), (800) 822-7422 (nationwide). This newsletter, available by free subscription (though donations are very welcome), reports on availability and usage of safe medical/pharmaceutical treatments and gives information on treatment strategies. Mostly written by the widely-respected activist Martin Delaney, *PI Perspective* also offers fascinating, critical commentary on the national approach to AIDS treatment issues.

Reports from the Holocaust, by Larry Kramer (New York, NY: St. Martin's Press, 1989). This is not a book that will lead you to a "serene" state of mind or in any way calm you, but it will contribute to your sense of courage growing out of anger, empowerment growing out of rage, and your rightful sense of righteous indignation—all components of a balanced acknowledgement of the issues and feelings surrounding AIDS. Over the years of the AIDS epidemic, Kramer has written numerous letters to the editor, articles about AIDS, political diatribes, and so on, and this book collects them into one volume. Reading them has the curious effect of angering and empowering you at the same time, because, after reading the pieces, you think to yourself, "Well, I really could do more. I really should do more. I really *can* do more. And my life probably depends on it." And that is very empowering, very inspiring. Don't read *Reports* if you're already dealing with too much anger or are feeling emotionally vulnerable. But if you're in a quandary about motivating yourself to do something about the epidemic beyond self-treatment, this book can be a powerful incentive to take action.

The Road Less Traveled, by M. Scott Peck, M.D. (New York, NY: Simon & Schuster, 1978). Reading this book is very comforting. After reading it, one feels really *good* about life, because Dr. Peck soothes worries, fears, anxieties, tensions—all the emotional tumbleweeds that inhibit happy living and restrict personal growth. The book shows how to confront your problems and work to resolve them, which is essentially what is meant by the "road less traveled," as most people tend to remain stuck in their old behavior patterns and habits, even if those patterns are making them miserable. Dr. Peck shows how to break out of that mold and tackle your problems with courage, patience, and resolve.

Strategies for Survival: A Gay Health Manual for the Age of AIDS, by Martin Delaney and Peter Goldblum, with Joseph Brewer (New York, NY: St. Martin's Press, 1987). This is a tremendously useful workbook for gay men, developed through several years of careful research. Not only is the book optimistic in tone, it is very sex-positive. By working your way through it, the book helps you to define those areas of your life where you need to make changes and improvements, so that rather than flounder in the dark, wondering what to do next, you can sit down with this workbook and "fill in the blanks" to help you reach the right decisions for your life—whether it's about treatment, safe sex, exercise, lifestyle, and so on.

Treatment Issues (The GMHC Newsletter of Experimental AIDS Therapies), published by Gay Men's Health Crisis, Department of Medical Information, 132 W. 24th Street, Box 274, New York, NY 10011. Rather more technical than other AIDS newsletters, this one reports ten times a year on various treatments, clinical trials, and AIDS resources. The writing is very dry, but I find the coverage to be thorough and reliably accurate, without optimism or pessimism.

When Bad Things Happen to Good People, by Harold S. Kushner (New York, NY: Schocken, 1981; Avon Books, 1983). Anyone who is troubled by the unfairness of AIDS and who is angry about having to deal with this awful epidemic will find much comfort and food for thought in this book. It was a bestseller when it came out. It presents a fresh and clear-minded approach to the reality of tragedy, illness, and death. Rabbi Kushner makes the strong point that when faced with personal tragedy, we should not ask the question "Why did this happen to me?" He shows that more often than not, there is no answer to that question, because there's simply no reason. Tragedy, illness, death—these are all random and natural parts of life, and we must learn to accept them as such. But beyond that, he says that asking such a question is clearly wrong-headed. Rather, we should ask, "Now that this has happened to me, what can I do about it?"

Working Inside Out, by Margo Adair (Berkeley, CA: Wingbow Press, 1985). In this book Margo Adair presents the techniques of relaxation, with a step-by-step guide on how to meditate. In addition to this book, Margo Adair has prepared cassette tapes of guided visualizations/meditations specifically for people with AIDS or for the worried well. For more information and an order form, contact: Tools for Change, Box 14141, San Francisco, CA 94114.

AIDS ORGANIZATIONS:

PROJECT INFORM
347 Dolores Street, Suite 301
San Francisco, CA 94110

National toll-free phone: (800) 822-7422
California toll-free phone: (800) 334-7422
Local phone: (415) 558-9051

Project Inform is an organization that provides information about alternative treatment approaches for AIDS, ARC, and HIV infection. If you want to find out more about treatment substances that many people are using, this is the place to contact. You can write or call them and ask for their information packet. You'll receive copies of basic information, medical reports, and referral numbers regarding safe and effective alternative/experimental treatments. You can request info packets for specific treatments as well. In addition, their staff is ready to answer questions and to provide additional referrals. This is a valuable organization, because it is one of the only places where you can get all this information in one place, easily and quickly. Trying to research the available alternative treatments can be painstaking and confusing. Project Inform has done most of that research for you, so the information is now readily available to the public.

AIDS FOUNDATIONS & HOTLINES:

Throughout the United States are many local AIDS foundations and health organizations that have telephone "hotlines" where individuals can call for further information, referrals, and, often, crisis counseling. Telephone information can usually find a hotline number in your area if you just call and ask for "AIDS Hotline," "AIDS Project," or "AIDS information." But if you can't find such an organization or number in your area, try calling the national AIDS hotline at (800) 342-2437. If you want immediate information about experimental drug trials, call the hotline of the AIDS Clinical Trials Information Service, toll-free at (800) 874-2572. Both the national AIDS hotline and the Clinical Trials Info Service have huge databases and can refer you to information resources and AIDS agencies in your area, or perhaps answer your questions directly.

ABOUT THE AUTHOR

P AUL REED is the author of two novels, *Longing* (1988) and *Facing It* (1984). He is the co-author of *How To Persuade Your Lover To Use a Condom . . . And Why You Should*. He has written for the national gay press, including *The Advocate* and the *Bay Area Reporter*. He holds an M.A. in cultural anthropology from the University of California, Davis. Mr. Reed makes his home in San Francisco.